THE
LOW-GL
DIET
COUNTER

Other Low-GL books by Patrick Holford:

The Low-GL Diet Bible
The Low-GL Diet Made Easy
The Low-GL Diet Cookbook
Food GLorious Food

patrick
HOLFORD

THE
LOW-GL
DIET
COUNTER

piatkus

PIATKUS

First published in Great Britain in 2006 by Piatkus Books
This expanded version first published 2011

Reprinted 2006, 2007, 2008, 2009 (twice), 2010, 2012

A CIP catalogue record for this book
is available from the British Library.

ISBN 978-0-7499-2678-6

Typeset in Minion by Phoenix Photosetting, Chatham, Kent
Printed and bound by
CPI Group (UK) Ltd, Croydon, CR0 4YY

Piatkus
An imprint of
Little, Brown Book Group
100 Victoria Embankment
London EC4Y 0DY

An Hachette UK Company
www.hachette.co.uk

www.piatkus.co.uk

Contents

Part **1**

GLs **Explained**

Introduction

This book is designed to help you make healthier choices when planning your meals and eating out. It accompanies my hugely successful books, *The Low-GL Diet Bible* and *The Low-GL Diet Cookbook*, helping you to put the advice into practice when planning meals, shopping for food or eating out. It works equally well on its own – for anyone trying to steer clear of refined, high-sugar foods – or as an aid to ensure that you are getting a balanced diet and/or losing weight.

GL or Glycemic Load – the backbone of my low-GL diet – is a tool that tells you exactly what a particular food or meal will do to your blood sugar. This is dietary gold dust, because your blood sugar levels are intimately connected with hunger, and so with how we eat.

GL is a much more accurate and practical tool than the well-known GI, or Glycemic Index. GI is a way of scoring how fast the carbohydrate within food raises your blood sugar compared with pure glucose – assessing its quality to show whether it is fast (bad) or slow (good) to release its sugar into the blood. GL goes one better than GI by factoring in the *quantity* as well as the *quality* of carbohydrate. This gives you a far more accurate reflection of the effect on your blood sugar. Take watermelon, for example, which contains fast-releasing sugar and therefore has a high GI of 72 (out of 100) – enough to put it out of bounds for any GI dieter. This is quite unnecessary, however, since on closer inspection we discover that only 6g of a 120g slice of watermelon contains this carbohydrate – most of it is actually water. From this we can work out an accurate GL score:

> **GI (divided by 100)**
> **x available carbohydrate (in grams) = GL**
>
> **For watermelon: 0.72 x 6g = 4.32**

So we can round this to 4 **GL**, a very low GL score, putting watermelon firmly on the Holford low-GL diet menu.

To put this in perspective:

- a GL of 10 or less is good;

- a GL of 11–14 is OK;

- a GL of 15 or more is bad.

However, even this is only a guide because the amount of a food you eat will obviously alter its effect on your blood sugar, and hence your weight. So, while generally I say liberally eat the good, low-GL foods (shown with a white background in the GL tables), limit the OK ones (grey background) and avoid the high ones (shown in white text on black) what is most important if you want to lose weight is to limit the total glycemic load of your diet.

Weight Loss

To lose weight the low-GL way, follow these simple rules:

- *eat* no more than 40 **GL** a day:
    - 10 **GL** each for breakfast, lunch and dinner,
    - 5 **GL** each for a morning and afternoon snack,
    - you can also have a further 5 **GL** for drinks – or the occasional pudding;

- always eat protein with carbohydrate;

- choose essential fats (omega-3 and omega-6 in oily fish, nuts and seeds) instead of saturated fats (in meat and dairy products).

This is how your GL allowance breaks down per day if you want to lose weight:

Daily GL allowance for weight loss

Breakfast	10 🇬🇱
Midmorning snack	5 🇬🇱
Lunch	10 🇬🇱
Midafternoon snack	5 🇬🇱
Dinner	10 🇬🇱
Additional points for drinks or puddings	5 🇬🇱
TOTAL	45 🇬🇱

You can find out the GL score of individual foods using this counter, making it easy to calculate the overall score of each meal. The charts show the serving size in grams or millilitres and what that looks like, plus the GL score per serving. You'll soon see that a bowl of oats, for example, has a very low GL score that fits the goal, whereas a sugar-coated cereal is much higher, making it easy for you to steer clear of the unhealthy options. Each section provides clear GL goals for each meal.

Once you have reached your target weight you can increase your overall GL intake by upping the carbohydrate serving size. See 'Maintain Your Weight' on page 20 for more details.

The Protein—Carb Connection

Protein helps to slow down the release of sugar from carbohydrates. Protein-rich foods such as eggs, meat, fish, dairy products, and nuts and seeds help us lose weight because they have virtually no effect on blood sugar, yet they fill us up. Standard high-protein diets make use of this advantage, but they can be problematic, particularly if they are based on a lot of animal protein such as dairy products and red meat, which are high in saturated fat and hormone residues from the animals, increasing risk of heart disease and cancer and disrupting our own hormonal systems. The healthiest solution is to eat protein with low-GL carbohydrates, not instead of them. That way you stabilise blood sugar, feel fuller for longer and lose weight, all without risking your health.

You need around 20g of protein at each meal. This is easy to achieve – the chart below shows you what this looks like on the plate:

How big is a protein serving?

Protein	Serving	
Tofu and tempeh	160g	¾ packet
Soya mince	100g	3 tbsp
Chicken (no skin)	50g	1 very small breast
Turkey (no skin)	50g	½ small breast
Quorn	120g	⅓ pack
Salmon and trout	55g	1 very small fillet
Tuna (canned in brine)	50g	¼ tin
Sardines (canned in brine)	75g	⅔ tin
Cod	65g	1 very small fillet
Clams	60g	¼ can
Prawns	85g	6 large prawns
Mackerel	85g	1 medium fillet
Oysters	–	15
Yoghurt (natural, low fat)	285g	½ a large tub
Cottage cheese	120g	½ a medium tub

chart continues ➤

Protein	Serving	
Hummus	200g	1 small tub
Skimmed milk	440ml	about ¾ pint
Soya milk	415ml	about ¾ pint
Eggs (boiled)	–	2
Quinoa	125g	1 large serving bowl
Baked beans	310g	¾ tin
Kidney beans	175g	⅓ tin
Black-eyed beans	175g	⅓ tin
Lentils	165g	⅓ tin

A Word on Fats

While fats themselves don't have any effect on blood sugar and as such are low-GL, the amount and type of fat you eat will still affect how much weight you lose – or put on for that matter! This means that you still need to monitor your fat intake – a fact ignored on classic low-carb diets.

Saturated fat (from animal products, in particular red meat and full-fat dairy products, and some nuts such as peanuts and cashews) is easily stored by the body as fat, not to mention clogging up arteries and raising LDL (low-density lipoprotein – or bad) cholesterol to increase your risk of stroke and heart disease.

Worse still are hydrogenated fats which are artificially produced by the food industry to increase shelf life of processed foods such as crisps, biscuits and ready meals. This not only is stored as fat, clogs up arteries and raises LDL cholesterol like saturated fats, but it also lowers HDL (high-density lipoprotein – or good) cholesterol, further increasing your risk of cardiovascular problems. Avoid any food that lists hydrogenated or partially hydrogenated oil in the ingredients list.

The partially hydrogenated oils are especially bad because they create a kind of damaged fat called a trans-fat. High temperature cooking, such as deep-frying, also creates these trans-fats which then damage the body and brain. So, fried, processed foods are a double whammy as far as your health is concerned.

Essential fats, however, are just as the name implies: crucial to our health. These are polyunsaturated fats and there are two types in particular that we must get from our diet, since we cannot make them ourselves.

Omega-3s

Found in oily fish such as salmon, tuna, trout, mackerel, sardines and anchovies, and in some nuts and seeds (such as flax and pumpkin seeds and walnuts and their oils), these polyunsaturated fats have myriad funct-ions: they help maintain a healthy weight by making hormone-like substances called prostaglandins, which help to control metabolism and our ability to burn fat; they also actively protect your heart and help produce smooth, supple skin to stave off wrinkles.

Omega-6s

Found in nuts and seeds (such as sunflower, sesame and pumpkin seeds and their oils, also starflower or safflower oil, evening primrose oil, corn oil and soya oil), these polyunsaturated fats help maintain hormone balance (reducing symptoms of PMS for example) and again ensure you have healthy skin.

It will come as no surprise, therefore, to hear that the fats recommended on the Holford low-GL diet are primarily the essential fats, with saturated fats limited and hydrogenated fats avoided entirely. This marks it out from old-fashioned low-fat diets, which avoided all fats indiscriminately, and classic low-carb diets, which do not restrict saturated fats.

To get enough essential fats, you need to pick two of any of the following options each day. Limit oily fish to three times a week (except tuna, which owing to its contamination with mercury should be an occasional treat no more than twice a month):

Breakfast: a dessertspoon of seeds (half pumpkin, half flax is excellent, or you can mix in some sesame and sunflower too) with your breakfast cereal or added to a smoothie such as my Get Up & Go Low GI/GL Shake. *The Low-GL Diet Cookbook* also has some delicious breakfast cereal recipes that include seeds.

Snacks: a dessertspoon of pumpkin seeds with a piece of fruit.

chart continues ➤

Main meals: a small serving of oily fish or a dessertspoon of pumpkin seeds.

Salad dressings: a dessertspoon of seed oil (available from good health-food stores – buy ones that are refrigerated to protect the delicate omega oils).

Personalise Your GL Allowance

While 45 **GL** per day is the average, what if you're tall or short, or very active? The table on page 20 shows you how to tailor-make your GL allowance to suit your build and lifestyle.

Height	Average exercise per day (mins)						
	0	15	30	45	60	90	120
5ft	35	35	40	45	45	50	55
5ft 3in	40	40	40	45	50	55	60
5ft 6in	40	40	40	45	50	55	60
5ft 9in	40	40	45	50	55	60	65
6ft	45	45	50	55	60	65	70
6ft 3in	50	50	55	60	65	70	75
6ft 6in	55	55	60	65	70	75	80

Maintain Your Weight

Once you have achieved your target weight, you can increase your daily GL intake to 65 (that is 15 **GL** at breakfast, lunch and supper, with two 5 GL snacks as before, and an additional 10 **GL** to have a drink, starter or pudding). This means you can increase your carbohydrate serving at each main meal.

On the next page is a breakdown of your new GL allowance each day to maintain weight.

Daily GL allowance for maintaining your ideal weight

Breakfast	15 GL
Midmorning snack	5 GL
Lunch	15 GL
Midafternoon snack	5 GL
Dinner	15 GL
Additional points for drinks or puddings	10 GL
TOTAL	**65 GL**

Here are a few sample menus to show you what this looks like:

Breakfast

Cereal (10 GL) with milk/yoghurt (0 GL) + fruit (5 GL) = 15 GL

Or thick slice of wholemeal toast (10 GL) with peanut butter (0 GL) plus a bowl of strawberries (5 GL) = 15 GL

Main meals

Pasta (10 **GL**) + pesto (2 **GL**) + roasted vegetables
(3 **GL**) = 15 **GL**

Or rice (10 **GL**) + fish fillet (0 **GL**) + steamed vegetables
(3 **GL**) = 13 **GL**

Note that this last example leaves you with 2 **GL** spare from the 15 GL allowance. You can therefore either increase the amount of vegetables you serve with the dish or perhaps serve them with a sauce. Alternatively, you can add the extra **GL** to your additional 10 **GL** per day for drinks, starters or pudding and indulge in the odd treat. (See my *Low-GL Diet Cookbook* for some fabulous puddings and teatime goodies that all fit the GL allowance, such as chocolate hazelnut mousse or an amazing lemon cheesecake for just 4 **GL**!)

Starters, drinks or puddings

With your extra 10 **GL** to enjoy once you have lost weight, you can increase your daily food intake to include a starter and a pudding at supper for example, or an extra glass of wine or fruit juice, as long as your treats don't exceed 10 Ⓖ per day. See *The Low-GL Diet Cookbook* for some enticing recipes to spend your extra points.

Part **2**

The GL Food Tables

Breakfast

The goal:

- eat no more than 10 **GL** to lose weight (or 15 **GL** to maintain your weight);

- combine protein with carbohydrate.

The best types of breakfast for weight loss are:

- *either* cereal with milk/yoghurt (5 **GL**) + fruit (5 **GL**) = 10 **GL**;

- *or* bread/baked item (10 **GL**) + egg/meat/fish/ (eg kippers) (0 **GL**) = 10 **GL**.

Protein foods such as dairy products have a minimal GL score, leaving you with 5 **GL** for cereal and another for fruit. Eggs, meat and fish contain virtually no carbohydrate at all, so they have a GL of 0, again leaving you with 10 **GL** for bread.

The lowest-GL choices are oat flakes or porridge made with milk or water, sprinkled with berries and ground mixed seeds (to provide essential fats – see page

17 for more information on the importance of good fats), or toasted rye or wholemeal bread with a poached egg, or try the delicious low-carb muesli with apple compote and yoghurt, or the low-GL granola with rhubarb compote and milk from *The Low-GL Diet Cookbook*.

Food	Goal
Bakery items	10
Bread	10
Breakfast cereals	5
Fruit	5
Dairy products and alternatives, eggs, meat, fish	0–3

KEY TO TABLES

White background: Low-GL foods

Grey background: Average foods (to be limited)

Black background: High-GL foods (to be avoided)

BREAKFASTS

GL rating	Food	Serving size in g	Looks like	GL per serving
	BAKERY PRODUCTS			
1	Low-carb muffin*	–	1 muffin	5
1	Muffin – apple, made without sugar	60	1 muffin	9
1	Waffles	35	half a waffle	10
2	Muffin – apple muffin, made with sugar	60	1 muffin	13
2	Crumpet	50	1 crumpet	13
2	Muffin – apple, oat, sultana, made from packet mix	50	1 muffin	14
3	Muffin – bran	57	1 muffin	15
3	Muffin – blueberry	57	1 muffin	17
3	Muffin – banana, oat and honey	50	1 muffin	17
3	Croissant	57	1 croissant	17
3	Muffin – carrot	57	1 muffin	20
3	Pop Tarts, double chocolate	50	quarter of a pop tart	25

table continues ➤

GL rating	Food	Serving size in g	Looks like	GL per serving
	BREADS			
1	Wheat bread, Burgen brand Burgen Soy-Lin, Kibbled Soy and Linseed	30	1½ slices	3
1	Wheat bread, Burgen brand Oat Bran and Honey Loaf with Barley	30	1½ slices	3
1	Rice bread, high-amylose	20	1 small slice	5
1	Rice bread, low-amylose	20	1 small slice	5
1	Wholemeal rye bread	20	1 thin slice	5
1	Rye kernel (pumpernickel) bread	30	1 slice	6
1	Sourdough rye	30	1 slice	6
1	Wheat bread, Vogel brand Honey and Oats	30	1 small slice	7
1	White, high-fibre	30	1 thick slice	9
1	Wholemeal (wholewheat) wheat-flour bread	30	1 thick slice	9
1	Gluten-free fibre-enriched	30	1 thick slice	9
1	Gluten-free multigrain bread	30	1 slice	10
1	Light rye	30	1 slice	10

GL rating	Food	Serving size in g	Looks like	GL per serving
1	White wheat-flour bread	30	1 slice	10
1	Pitta bread, white	30	1 pitta	10
1	Wheat-flour flatbread	30	1 slice	10
2	Gluten-free white bread	30	1 slice	11
3	Baguette, white, plain	30	⅓ baton	15
3	Bagel, white, frozen	70	1 bagel	25
	BREAKFAST CEREALS			
1	Porridge made from rolled oats	30	large bowl	2
1	Low-GL granola*	–	1 large serving	3.5
1	Low-carb muesli*	–	1 serving	4
1	Low-carb granola (GoodCarb Original)	50	medium bowl	5
1	Granola, Belgian Chocolate, Goodcarb	50	1 medium serving	6
1	Granola, Cinnamon and Apple, Goodcarb	50	1 medium serving	6
1	All-Bran (Kellogg's)	30	1 small serving	6
1	Granola, Treacle and Pecan, Goodcarb	50	a small serving	7
1	Muesli, gluten-free	30	1 medium serving	7

table continues ➤

GL rating	Food	Serving size in g	Looks like	GL per serving
1	Get Up & Go with strawberries and ½ pint milk E	30	½ pint drink	8.5
1	Cinnamon apple porridge with milk*	–	1 serving	10
1	Low-carb muesli with berries and cow's/soya/nut milk*	–	1 serving	10
1	Muesli (Alpen)	30	1 serving	10
1	Muesli, natural	30	1 serving	10
2	Weetabix	25	2 biscuits	11
2	Raisin Bran (Kellogg's)	30	1 medium serving	12
2	Bran Flakes	30	1 medium serving	13
2	Sultana Bran (Kellogg's)	30	1 medium serving	14
2	Special K (Kellogg's)	30	1 medium serving	14
3	Cheerios (Nestlé)	30	1 medium serving	15
3	Frosties, sugar-coated cornflakes (Kellogg's)	30	1 medium serving	15
3	Grapenuts (Kraft Foods)	30	1 medium serving	15
3	Golden Wheats (Kellogg's)	30	1 medium serving	16
3	Puffed Wheat	30	1 medium serving	16

GL rating	Food	Serving size in g	Looks like	GL per serving
3	Honey Smacks (Kellogg's)	30	1 medium serving	16
3	Cornflakes, Crunchy Nut (Kellogg's)	30	1 medium serving	17
3	Shredded Wheat	40	2 biscuits	20
3	Coco Pops (cocoa-flavoured puffed rice)	30	1 medium serving	20
3	Rice Krispies (Kellogg's)	30	1 medium serving	21
3	Cornflakes (Kellogg's)	30	1 medium serving	21

DAIRY PRODUCTS AND ALTERNATIVES

GL rating	Food	Serving size in g	Looks like	GL per serving
1	Hazelnut yoghurt*	–	1 serving	2
1	Plain yoghurt (no sugar)	200	1 small pot	3
1	Non-fat yoghurt (plain, no sugar)	200	1 small pot	3
1	Milk, full-fat, in ml	250	1 glass	3
1	Milk, skim (Canada), in ml	250	1 glass	4
1	Soya yoghurt (Provamel)	200	1 large bowl	7
1	Soya milk (no sugar), in ml	250	1 glass	7
1	Custard, homemade from milk	100	1½ small cups	7

table continues ➤

GL rating	Food	Serving size in g	Looks like	GL per serving
1	Low-fat yoghurt, fruit, sugar, (Ski)	150	1 small pot	7.5
1	Soya milk (sweetened with apple juice concentrate), in ml	250	1 glass	8
1	Soya milk, reduced-fat (1.5%), 120mg calcium, in ml	250	1 glass	8
1	Soya milk (sweetened with sugar), in ml	250	1 glass	9
1	Ice cream, regular	60	2 scoops	10
2	Rice milk, E, in ml	250	1 glass	14
3	Milk, condensed, sweetened (Nestlé), in ml	50	1 dessertspoon	17
	FRUIT AND FRUIT PRODUCTS			
1	Blackberries E	120	1 medium bowl	1
1	Blueberries E	120	1 medium bowl	1
1	Raspberries E	120	1 medium bowl	1
1	Strawberries, fresh, raw	120	1 medium bowl	1
1	Cherries, raw, not stoned	120	1 medium bowl	3

GL rating	Food	Serving size in g	Looks like	GL per serving
1	Grapefruit, raw	120	½ medium	3
1	Pear, raw	120	1 medium	4
1	Plum yoghurt crunch*	–	1 medium serving	4
1	Melon, eg cantaloupe, raw	120	½ small	4
1	Watermelon, raw	120	1 medium slice	4
1	Apple compote*	–	1 serving	5
1	Peaches raw (or canned in natural juice)	120	1	5
1	Apricots, raw	120	4 apricots	5
1	Oranges, raw	120	1 large	5
1	Plums, raw	120	4	5
1	Apples, raw	120	1 small	6
1	Kiwi fruit, raw	120	1	6
1	Pineapple, raw	120	1 medium slice	7
1	Grapes, raw	120	16	8
1	Mango, raw	120	1½ slices	8
1	Apricots, dried	60	6 apricots	9
1	Fruit cocktail, canned (Delmonte)	120	small can	9
1	Pawpaw/papaya, raw	120	½ small papaya	10

table continues ➤

GL rating	Food	Serving size in g	Looks like	GL per serving
1	Prunes, pitted	60	6 prunes	10
1	Apple, dried	60	6 rings	10
2	Banana, raw	120	1 small	12
2	Apricots, canned in light syrup	120	1 small tin	12
3	Lychees, canned in syrup and drained	120	1 small tin	16
3	Figs, dried, tenderised, (Dessert Maid)	60	3	16
3	Sultanas	60	30	25
3	Raisins	60	30	28
3	Dates, dried	60	8	42
	JAMS/SPREADS			
1	Pumpkin seed butter E	16	1 tbsp	1
1	Peanut butter (no sugar) E	16	1 tbsp	1
1	Blueberry spread (no sugar) E	10	1 dessertspoon	1
1	Apricot fruit spread, reduced-sugar	10	1 dessertspoon	2

GL rating	Food	Serving size in g	Looks like	GL per serving
1	Orange marmalade	10	1 dessertspoon	3
1	Strawberry jam	10	1 dessertspoon	3
	PROTEIN FOODS			
1	Sardines (canned)	75	⅔ can	0
1	Eggs (boiled)	–	2 medium	0
1	Boiled egg and soldiers*	–	1 serving	9
1	Scrambled eggs on toast*	–	1 serving	9
1	Smoked trout omelette with 1½ slices of rye bread*	–	1 serving	9
2	Smoked salmon and chive scrambled eggs with 1 toasted pitta*	–	1 serving	11
2	Baked beans, canned	310	¾ can	14

* These items appear in *The Low-GL Diet Cookbook*
All dishes marked E have estimated GL scores

Snacks

The goal:

- eat no more than 5 **GL** per snack;

- have a snack midmorning and another midafternoon;

- combine protein with carbohydrate.

GL-friendly snacks include:

- fruit (5 **GL**) + nuts (0 **GL**) = 5 **GL**;

- bread/oat cakes (5 **GL**) + protein-rich spread (eg peanut butter, hummus, egg mayo) (0 **GL**) = 5 **GL**;

- crudités (eg carrot and baby corn) (5 **GL**) + protein-rich dip (eg hummus, cottage cheese) (0 **GL**) = 5 **GL**.

You can eat a small apple or pear or a punnet of berries for 5 **GL**, whereas bananas and dried fruit have a much higher GL.

You'll also see that rye bread has a much lower GL than standard wheat bread, so you can eat a whole slice of pumpernickel or sourdough rye bread for 5 ⓖⓛ but only half a slice of normal bread. Oat cakes are another low-GL snack – you can have 2½ rough oat cakes for 5 ⓖⓛ.

Again, protein foods such as peanut butter and hummus, or nuts, contain negligible ⓖⓛ.

Food	Goal
Bread/crackers	5
Fruit	5
Nuts	0–1
Dips or spreads	0–1

SNACKS

GL rating	Food	Serving size in g	Looks like	GL per serving
	BAKERY PRODUCTS			
1	Low-carb muffin*	–	1 muffin	5
1	Apple and almond cake*	–	1 medium slice	5
1	Carrot and walnut cake*	–	1 medium slice	5
1	Scones, plain, made from packet mix	25	small scone	7
1	Muffin – apple, made without sugar	60	1 muffin	9
2	Muffin – apple muffin, made with sugar	60	1 muffin	13
2	Crumpet	50	1 crumpet	13
2	Muffin – apple, oat, sultana, made from packet mix	50	1 muffin	14
3	Muffin – bran	57	1 muffin	15
3	Banana cake, made without sugar	80	1 medium slice	16
3	Muffin – blueberry	57	1 muffin	17
3	Muffin – banana, oat and honey	50	1 muffin	17

GL rating	Food	Serving size in g	Looks like	GL per serving
3	Croissant	57	1 croissant	17
3	Doughnut	47	1 plain doughnut	17
3	Sponge cake, plain	63	1 slice	17
3	Muffin – carrot	57	1 muffin	20
3	Chocolate cake (packet mix) + frosting, Betty Crocker	111	quarter of a slice	20
	BREADS			
1	Wheat bread, Burgen brand Burgen Soy-Lin, Kibbled Soy and Linseed	30	1½ slices	3
1	Wheat bread, Burgen brand Oat Bran and Honey Loaf with Barley	30	1½ slices	3
1	Volkenbrot, wholemeal rye bread	20	1 slice	5
1	Rice bread, high-amylose	20	1 small slice	5
1	Rice bread, low-amylose	20	1 small slice	5
1	Wholemeal rye bread	20	1 thin slice	5
1	Wheat tortilla (Mexican)	30	1 tortilla	5
1	Chapatti, white wheat flour, thin	30	1 chapatti	5

table continues ➤

GL rating	Food	Serving size in g	Looks like	GL per serving
1	Rye kernel (pumpernickel) bread	30	1 slice	6
1	Sourdough rye	30	1 slice	6
1	Wheat bread, Vogel brand Honey and Oats	30	1 small slice	7
1	White, high-fibre	30	1 thick slice	9
1	Wholemeal (wholewheat) wheat flour bread	30	1 thick slice	9
1	Gluten-free fibre-enriched	30	1 thick slice	9
1	Gluten-free multigrain bread	30	1 slice	10
1	Light rye	30	1 slice	10
1	White wheat flour bread	30	1 slice	10
1	Pitta bread, white	30	1 pitta	10
1	Wheat flour flatbread	30	1 slice	10
2	Gluten-free white bread	30	1 slice	11
2	Corn tortilla	50	1 tortilla	12
3	Middle Eastern flatbread	30	1 slice	15
3	Baguette, white, plain	30	1/3 baton	15
3	Bagel, white, frozen	70	1 bagel	25

GL rating	Food	Serving size in g	Looks like	GL per serving
	CRISPBREADS/CRACKERS			
1	Rough Oatcakes (Nairn's)	10	1 oat cake	2
1	Fine Oatcakes (Nairn's)	9	1 oat cake	3
1	Cheese Oatcakes (Nairn's)	8	1 oat cake	3
2	Cream cracker	25	2 biscuits	11
2	Rye crispbread	25	2 biscuits	11
2	Ryvita	–	half a cracker	11
3	Water cracker	25	3 biscuits	17
3	Puffed rice cakes	25	3 biscuits	17
3	Corn thins, puffed corn cakes	–	quarter of a cracker	18
	DAIRY PRODUCTS AND ALTERNATIVES			
1	Plain yoghurt (no sugar)	200	1 small pot	3
1	Non-fat yoghurt (plain, no sugar)	200	1 small pot	3
1	Cheese platter*	–	1 serving	6
1	Soya yoghurt (Provamel)	200	1 large bowl	7
1	Soya milk (no sugar), in ml	250	1 glass	7
1	Low-fat yoghurt, fruit, sugar (Ski)	150	1 small pot	7.5

table continues ➤

GL rating	Food	Serving size in g	Looks like	GL per serving
	FRUIT AND FRUIT PRODUCTS			
1	Blackberries E	120	1 medium bowl	1
1	Blueberries E	120	1 medium bowl	1
1	Raspberries E	120	1 medium bowl	1
1	Strawberries, fresh, raw	120	1 medium bowl	1
1	Cherries, raw, not stoned	120	1 medium bowl	3
1	Grapefruit, raw	120	½ medium	3
1	Pear, raw	120	1 medium	4
1	Melon, eg cantaloupe, raw	120	½ small	4
1	Watermelon, raw	120	1 medium slice	4
1	Peaches E	87	1 large	4
1	Apricots, raw	120	4 apricots	5
1	Nectarine E	136	1 nectarine	5
1	Oranges, raw	120	1 large	5
1	Plums, raw	120	4	5
1	Apples, raw	120	1 small	6
1	Kiwi fruit, raw	120	1	6
1	Pineapple, raw	120	1 medium slice	7
1	Grapes, raw	120	16	8

GL rating	Food	Serving size in g	Looks like	GL per serving
1	Mango, raw	120	1½ slices	8
1	Dried fruit leather, Windsor Farm Foods	30	three-quarters of a bar	8
1	Apricots, dried	60	6 apricots	9
1	Fruit cocktail, canned (Delmonte)	120	small can	9
1	Pawpaw/papaya, raw	120	½ small papaya	10
1	Prunes, pitted	60	6 prunes	10
1	Apple, dried	60	6 rings	10
2	Banana, raw	120	1 small	12
2	Apricots, canned in light syrup	120	1 small tin	12
3	Lychees, canned in syrup and drained	120	1 small tin	16
3	Figs, dried, tenderised (Dessert Maid)	60	3	16
3	Sultanas	60	30	25
3	Raisins	60	30	28
3	Dates, dried	60	8	42

table continues ➤

GL rating	Food	Serving size in g	Looks like	GL per serving
	JAMS/SPREADS			
1	Pumpkin seed butter E	16	1 tablespoon	1
1	Peanut butter (no sugar) E	16	1 tablespoon	1
1	Blueberry spread (no sugar) E	10	1 dessertspoon	1
1	Apricot fruit spread, reduced sugar	10	1 dessertspoon	2
1	Orange marmalade	10	1 dessertspoon	3
1	Strawberry jam	10	1 dessertspoon	3
1	Nutella, chocolate hazelnut spread	20	1 dessertspoon	4
	SNACK FOODS (SAVOURY)			
1	Guacamole*	–	1 serving	1
1	Olives, in brine E	50	7	1
1	Peanuts	50	2 medium handfuls	1
1	Yoghurt satay dip*	–	1 serving	1
1	Avocado and cream cheese dip*	–	1 serving	2
1	Tahini dip*	–	1 serving	2
1	Tamari toasted nuts*	–	1 serving	2
1	Cashew nuts, salted	50	2 medium handfuls	3

GL rating	Food	Serving size in g	Looks like	GL per serving
1	Potato crisps, plain, salted	30	1 small packet	7
1	Oat Bakes, Nairns	30	1 packet	9
1	Popcorn, salted, no sugar	25	1 small packet	10
3	Pretzels, oven-baked, traditional wheat flavour	30	15	16
3	Corn chips plain, salted	50	18	17
	SNACK FOODS (SWEET)			
1	Low-carb chocolate brownie (GoodCarb Real Belgian, all 3 flavours)	45	1 bar	3
1	Almond shortbread*	–	1 serving	4
1	Chocolate-dipped nuts*	–	1 serving	4
1	Oat Biscuits, Nairns	–	1 biscuit	4
1	Apple cereal bar (Fruitus) E	35	1	5
1	Marzipan truffles*	–	1 serving	5
1	Fruit and veg bar (Rebar) E	50	1	8
2	Muesli bar containing dried fruit	30	1	13
2	Chocolate, white (Milky Bar: Nestlé)	50	third of a bar	13
2	Chocolate, milk, plain (Nestlé)	50	third of a bar	14

table continues ➤

GL rating	Food	Serving size in g	Looks like	GL per serving
2	Apricot fruit bar (dried apricot filling in wholemeal pastry)	35	1	17
3	Twix caramel cookie bar (M&M/Mars, USA)	60	1 bar (2 fingers)	17
3	Snickers Bar	60	1	19
3	Polos – peppermint sweets	30	16	21
3	Jellybeans, assorted colours	30	9	22
3	Pop Tarts, double choc	50	1	24
3	Mars Bar	60	1	26
	PROTEIN FOODS			
1	Eggs (boiled)	–	2 medium	0
1	Cottage cheese	120	½ medium tub	2
1	Egg mayonnaise	120	½ medium tub	2
1	Hummus	200	1 small tub	6

* These items appear in *The Low-GL Diet Cookbook*
All dishes marked E have estimated GL scores

Main Meals

The goal:

- eat no more than 10 **GL** at lunch and supper to lose weight (or 15 **GL** to maintain your weight);

- combine protein with carbohydrate at each meal.

The GL guide for main meals is as follows:

Starchy vegetables/carbohydrates (eg rice, pasta, potatoes) (7 **GL**) + non-starchy vegetables (eg broccoli, salad) (3 **GL**) + protein (eg chicken, fish, tofu) (0 **GL**) = 10 **GL**.

The chart below shows you exactly how much of common carbohydrate foods, including starchy vegetables, you can eat for 7 **GL**:

Starchy Carb Servings   7 **GL**
                            (uncooked weight)

Pumpkin/squash	185g
Carrot	160g
Swede	150g

chart continues ➤

Beetroot	110g
Boiled potato	3 small potatoes (75g)
Quinoa	65g
Cornmeal	60g
Corn on the cob	½ a cob (60g)
Baked potato	½ a baked potato (60g)
Sweet potato	½ a sweet potato (60g)
French fries	50g
Brown basmati rice	45g
Pearl barley	45g
Wholemeal pasta	40g
Brown rice	35g
Starchy Carb Servings	**7 GL**
White pasta	35g
Broad beans	30g
Couscous	25g
White rice	25g

When combining legumes such as chickpeas and beans with other starchy vegetables/carbohydrates such as rice and pasta, bear in mind that legumes contain carbohydrate as well as protein, so you need to halve the amount of starchy veg/carbohydrate serving size from 7 **GL** to 3.5 **GL**.

Don't forget that quinoa is a good source of protein as well as carbohydrate, so you use it as protein and/or carbohydrate in a dish.

Example vegetarian meals include:

- starchy vegetables/carbohydrates (eg rice, pasta, potatoes, quinoa) (7 **GL**) + non-starchy vegetables (eg broccoli, salad) (3 **GL**) + protein (eg tofu, eggs) (0 **GL**) = 10 **GL**;

- quinoa (contains complete protein) (7 **GL**) + non-starchy vegetables (3 **GL**) = 10 **GL**;

- starchy vegetables/carbohydrates (eg rice) (3.5 **GL**) + non-starchy vegetables (eg broccoli, salad) (3 **GL**) + legumes (eg lentils, chickpeas) (3.5 GLs) = 10 **GL**.

Food	Goal
Starchy veg/grains (bread, rice, pasta, potatoes, legumes)	7
Non-starchy veg (salad, broccoli, peppers, green leafy veg, etc)	3
Protein (egg, meat, fish, tofu)	0–3
Legumes (eaten as protein with 3.5 ⓖⓛ rice or other starchy veg)	3.5

If you are used to cooking carbohydrate-heavy dishes such as spaghetti bolognaise, chilli with mounds of rice or leek and potato soup, take a look at *The Low-GL Diet Cookbook* for some suggestions and recipes with which to make over your favourite meals the low-GL way. All the old favourites, including the above examples, feature in the recipes, subtly tweaked to lower the GL score without compromising on flavour.

MAIN MEALS

GL rating	Food	Serving size in g	Looks like	GL per serving
	BREADS			
1	Sesame cornbread*	–	1 serving	1
1	Wheat bread, Burgen brand Burgen Soy-Lin, Kibbled Soy and Linseed	30	1½ slices	3
1	Wheat bread, Burgen brand Oat Bran and Honey Loaf with Barley	30	1½ slices	3
1	Rice bread, high-amylose	20	1 small slice	5
1	Rice bread, low-amylose	20	1 small slice	5
1	Wholemeal rye bread	20	1 thin slice	5
1	Wheat tortilla (Mexican)	30	1 tortilla	5
1	Chapatti, white wheat flour, thin	30	1 chapatti	5
1	Rye kernel (pumpernickel) bread	30	1 slice	6
1	Sourdough rye	30	1 slice	6
1	Wheat bread, Vogel brand Honey and Oats	30	1 small slice	7
1	White, high-fibre	30	1 thick slice	9

table continues ➤

GL rating	Food	Serving size in g	Looks like	GL per serving
1	Wholemeal (wholewheat) wheat-flour bread	30	1 thick slice	9
1	Gluten-free fibre-enriched	30	1 thick slice	9
1	Gluten-free multigrain bread	30	1 slice	10
1	Light rye	30	1 slice	10
1	White wheat flour bread	30	1 slice	10
1	Pitta bread, white	30	1 pitta	10
1	Wheat flour flatbread	30	1 slice	10
2	Gluten-free white bread	30	1 slice	11
2	Corn tortilla	50	1 tortilla	12
3	Middle Eastern flatbread	30	1 slice	15
3	Baguette, white, plain	30	⅓ baton	15
3	Bagel, white, frozen	70	1 bagel	25
	CEREAL GRAINS			
1	Semolina, cooked	150	1 large serving	6
1	Taco shells, cornmeal-based, baked (Old El Paso)	20	2 shells	8
1	Quinoa, boiled	150	1 large serving	8
1	Cornmeal, cooked	150	1 large serving	9

GL rating	Food	Serving size in g	Looks like	ⓖⓛ per serving
1	Kamut E, boiled	150	1 large serving	9
2	Pearl barley, boiled	150	1 medium serving	11
2	Cracked wheat (bulgur/bourghul), boiled	150	1 medium serving	12
2	Brown basmati rice, boiled	150	1 medium serving	13
3	Buckwheat, boiled	150	1 medium serving	16
3	Rice, brown, boiled	150	1 large serving	18
3	Long-grain, white, precooked microwaved 2 min. (Express Rice, Uncle Ben's)	150	1 medium serving	19
3	Basmati, white, boiled	150	1 medium serving	22
3	Couscous, boiled	150	1 medium serving	23
3	Rice, white, boiled	150	1 medium serving	23
3	Long-grain, boiled	150	1 medium serving	23
3	Millet, porridge	150	1 large serving	25
	CRISPBREADS/CRACKERS			
1	Rough Oatcakes (Nairn's)	10	1 oat cake	2
1	Fine Oatcakes (Nairn's)	9	1 oat cake	3
1	Cheese Oatcakes (Nairn's)	8	1 oat cake	3

table continues ➤

GL rating	Food	Serving size in g	Looks like	GL per serving
2	Cream cracker	25	2 biscuits	11
2	Rye crispbread	25	2 biscuits	11
3	Melba toast	30	third of a cracker	16
3	Water cracker	25	3 biscuits	17
3	Puffed rice cakes	25	3 biscuits	17
	LEGUMES AND NUTS			
1	Soya beans	150	²/₃ 410g can, drained	1
1	Peas, dried, boiled	150	½ cup	2
1	Spicy Mexican bean dip*	–	1 large serving	4
1	Pinto beans, boiled in salted water	150	²/₃ 410g can, drained	4
1	Borlotti beans, boiled, canned	150	²/₃ 410g can, drained	4
1	Hummus	100	½ small tub	5
1	Lentils	150	²/₃ 410g can, drained	5
1	Butter beans	150	²/₃ 410g can, drained	6
1	Split peas, yellow, boiled 20 min.	150	²/₃ cup	6
1	Lentil dahl*	–	large serving	7
1	Baked beans, canned	150	²/₃ can	7

GL rating	Food	Serving size in g	Looks like	GL per serving
1	Kidney beans	150	⅔ 410g can, drained	7
1	Borlotti bolognese*	–	1 serving	7
1	Chickpea curry*	–	1 serving	7
1	Chickpeas (garbanzo beans, Bengal gram), boiled	150	1 cup	8
1	Chestnuts, cooked E	150	¾ can	8
1	Flageolet beans, canned in brine E	150	⅔ 410g can, drained	8
1	Chickpeas, canned in brine	150	⅔ 410g can, drained	9
2	Haricot/Navy beans	150	⅔ 410g can, drained	12
2	Black-eyed beans, boiled	150	⅔ 410g can, drained	13
	PASTA AND NOODLES			
1	Lasagne, Dreamfields	56	1 serving	5
1	Macaroni, Dreamfields	56	1 serving	5
1	Penne, Dreamfields	56	1 serving	5
1	Spaghetti, Dreamfields	56	1 serving	5
1	Ravioli, durum wheat flour, meat filled, boiled	90	1 medium serving	7.5
1	Vermicelli, white, boiled	90	1 medium serving	8

table continues ➤

GL rating	Food	Serving size in g	Looks like	GL per serving
1	Spaghetti, wholemeal, boiled	90	1 medium serving	8
1	Pasta, wholemeal, boiled	90	1 medium serving	8
1	Fettuccine, egg	90	1 medium serving	9
1	Spirali, durum wheat, white, boiled to *al dente* texture	90	1 medium serving	9
1	Spaghetti, white, boiled	90	1 medium serving	9
1	Instant noodles	90	1 medium serving	9
1	Spaghetti, durum wheat, boiled 10–15 min.	90	1 medium serving	10
2	Gluten-free pasta, maize starch, boiled 8 min.	90	1 medium serving	11
2	Macaroni, plain	90	1 medium serving	11
2	Rice noodles, dried, boiled	90	1 medium serving	11
3	Udon noodles, plain, (buckwheat/wheat)	90	1 medium serving	15
3	Corn pasta, gluten-free (62.5g serving size)	–	1 medium serving	16
3	Gnocchi	90	1 medium serving	16
3	Rice pasta, brown, boiled 16 min.	90	1 medium serving	17
3	Linguine, thin, durum wheat	180	1 very small serving	23

GL rating	Food	Serving size in g	Looks like	GL per serving
	SOUPS			
1	Oriental chicken broth*	–	1 large serving	3
1	Thai mushroom broth*	–	1 serving	4
1	Tomato	250	½ can (1 serving)	6
1	Minestrone	250	½ can (1 serving)	7
1	Smoked mackerel, leek and bean soup*	–	small serving	7
1	Avocado gazpacho*	–	1 serving	8
1	Lentil, canned	250	½ can (1 serving)	9
2	Leek and potato*	–	1 serving	11
2	Chestnut and butterbean soup*	–	1 serving	12
3	Split-pea	250	½ can (1 serving)	16
3	Black-bean	250	½ can (1 serving)	17
3	Green-pea, canned	250	½ can (1 serving)	17
	VEGETABLES			
1	Aubergine E	100	½ small	1
1	Broccoli E	100	1 handful	1
1	Cabbage E	100	1 handful	1

table continues ➤

GL rating	Food	Serving size in g	Looks like	GL per serving
1	Cauliflower E	100	1 handful	1
1	Courgette E	100	1 small	1
1	Cucumber E	100	½ small	1
1	Lettuce E	100	large handful	0–1
1	Radish E	25	1 handful	1
1	Spinach E	100	large handful	1
1	Kale E	75	1 handful	1
1	Avocado E	190	1 medium	1
1	Leeks E	100	1 medium	1
1	Green beans E	75	1 handful	1
1	Tomato E	70	1 medium	2
1	Onion E	180	1 medium	2
1	Asparagus E	125	1 handful	2
1	Red pepper and cucumber salsa*	–	1 serving	2
1	Cauliflower dahl*	–	1 serving	2
1	Carrots	80	1 small	3
1	Green peas	80	1½ tbsp	3
1	Pumpkin/squash	80	1 serving	3

GL rating	Food	Serving size in g	Looks like	ⒼⓁ per serving
1	Cashew cauliflower cheese*	–	1 serving	3
1	Beetroot	80	2 small	5
1	Avocado potato salad*	–	1 serving	5
1	Roasted vegetables*	–	1 serving	5
1	Swede	150	⅓ swede	7
1	Sweet potato wedges*	–	small serving	8
1	Banana/plantain, green	120	1 very small	8
1	Broad beans	80	2 tbsp	9
1	Sweet potato and carrot mash*	–	1 serving	10
2	Parsnips	80	1 medium	12
2	Sweetcorn, on the cob, boiled	150	third of a cob of corn	14
2	Yam	150	1 medium	13
2	Boiled potato	150	3 small	14
2	Microwaved potato	150	3 small	14
3	Mashed potato	150	3 tbsp	15
3	New potato, unpeeled and boiled 20 min.	150	3 small	16
3	Instant mashed potato	150	3 tbsp	17

table continues ➤

GL rating	Food	Serving size in g	Looks like	GL per serving
3	Sweet potato	150	1 large	17
3	Baked potato, white, baked in skin	150	1 large	18
3	French fries	150	20	22
	PROTEIN FOODS			
1	Tofu and tempeh	160	¾ packet	0
1	Soya mince	100	3 tbsp	0
1	Chicken (no skin)	50	1 small breast	0
1	Turkey (no skin)	50	½ small breast	0
1	Quorn	120	⅓ pack	0
1	Salmon	55	1 small fillet	0
1	Trout	55	1 small fillet	0
1	Tuna (canned)	50	¼ tin	0
1	Sardines (canned)	75	⅔ can	0
1	Cod	65	1 small fillet	0
1	Prawns	85	6 large	0
1	Mackerel	85	1 medium fillet	0
1	Oysters	–	15	0
1	Eggs (boiled)	–	2 medium	0

GL rating	Food	Serving size in g	Looks like	GL per serving
1	Cottage cheese	120	½ medium tub	2
1	Egg mayonnaise	120	½ medium tub	2
1	Non-fat yoghurt (plain, no sugar)	285	½ large tub	4
1	Hummus	200	1 small tub	6
1	Lentils	165	⅓ tin	6
1	Milk, skim (Canada), in ml	440	large glass	7
1	Quinoa, boiled	125	large bowl	7
1	Kidney beans	175	⅓ tin	8
2	Baked beans, canned	310	¾ can	14
2	Black-eyed beans, boiled	175	⅓ tin	14
	COMPLETE DISHES			
1	Grilled trout with lemon and almonds*	–	1 serving	1
1	Nick's beefburgers*	–	2 burgers	1
1	Pesto-crusted salmon*	–	1 serving	1
1	Roast pepper and feta stuffed chicken*	–	1 serving	1
1	Spiced turkey burgers*	–	2 burgers	1
1	Teriyaki chicken*	–	1 serving	1

table continues ➤

GL rating	Food	Serving size in g	Looks like	GL per serving
1	Teriyaki salmon*	–	1 serving	1
1	Trout en papillote with lemon and garlic*	–	1 serving	1
1	Hot smoked salmon with crème fraiche and herb sauce*	–	1 serving	2
1	Lemon and coriander chicken en papillote*	–	1 serving	2
1	Greek salad*	–	1 serving	3
1	Chicken curry*	–	1 serving	3
1	Chicken with cherry tomatoes and crème fraiche*	–	1 serving	4
1	Halloumi kebabs*	–	2 skewers	4
1	Red lentil and smoked mackerel kedgeree*	–	1 serving	4
1	Salmon and cherry tomato bake*	–	1 serving	4
1	Teriyaki tofu*	–	1 serving	4
1	Venison sausage and mixed pepper casserole*	–	1 serving	4
1	Oriental broth, such as Tom Yum soup E	–	small bowl	4

GL rating	Food	Serving size in g	Looks like	ⓖⓛ per serving
1	Moussaka*	–	1 serving	5
1	Antipasti skewers*	–	1 serving	5
1	Chicken with aubergine and peppers*	–	1 serving	5
1	Greek salad skewers*	–	1 serving	5
1	Seafood souffle pie*	–	1 serving	5
1	Tuna steak with sesame quinoa*	–	1 serving	5
1	Sushi E	–	2 pieces fish on rice	5
1	Cashew and sesame quinoa*	–	1 serving	6
1	Hot smoked trout with pumpkin seed pesto and watercress open sandwich*	–	1 serving	6
1	Vegetable chilli*	–	1 serving	6
1	Bresaola and artichoke hearts on rye*	–	1 serving	7
1	Salad nicoise*	–	1 serving	7
1	Smoked mackerel salad*	–	1 serving	7
1	Creamy salmon with leeks*	–	1 serving	8
1	Mediterranean tomato risotto with tuna*	–	1 serving	8

table continues ➤

GL rating	Food	Serving size in g	Looks like	GL per serving
1	Poached haddock with cannellini bean mash*	–	1 serving	8
1	Stuffed peppers*	–	1 serving	9
1	Chicken curry with brown basmati rice*	–	medium plate	10
1	Teriyaki chicken with brown basmati rice*	–	medium plate	10
1	Chicken satay wrap*	–	1 wrap	10
1	Chilli con carne with quinoa*	–	medium plate	10
1	Hot smoked trout with flageolet beans in white sauce*	–	1 serving	10
1	Roasted chickpea and lemon tabboulleh*	–	1 serving	10
1	Sesame chicken and soba noodle steam-fry*	–	1 serving	10
2	Bangers and mash*	–	medium plate	11
2	Spaghetti bolognaise*	–	large plate	11
2	Mediterranean pasta*	–	small plate	11
2	Roasted pepper and artichoke tortilla*	–	1 serving	11
3	Chilli con carne with brown basmati rice*	–	large plate	15

GL rating	Food	Serving size in g	Looks like	GL per serving
3	Pasta with pesto	200	large plate	18
3	Pizza (thin base) E	150	large slice	18
3	Lasagne E	420	large serving	20
3	Cheeseburger E	130	medium	25
3	Hamburger E	120	medium	25
3	Fish/meat teriyaki/yakitori with white rice E	500	large serving	25
3	Fish/chicken satay (peanut sauce) with white rice E	320	medium serving	26
3	Meat curry (cream-based sauce, eg korma, masala) with white rice E	500	large serving	28
3	Meat curry (tomato-based sauce eg madras, rogan josh) with white rice E	500	large serving	28
3	Stir-fried meat/vegetables with white rice E	350	large serving	28
3	Meat/egg fried rice/noodles E	350	large serving	29
3	Pizza (thick base) E	300	large slice	36

* These items appear in *The Low-GL Diet Cookbook*
All dishes marked E have estimated GL scores

Puddings

The goal:

- have no more than 5 ⑤ for pudding.

If this seems difficult, look out for the dishes in the chart below marked with an asterisk to indicate that they feature in *The Low-GL Diet Cookbook*. All of which fit within the rules for low-GL puddings and are all naturally low in saturated fat and sugar. As a general guide, fruit- and protein-based puddings (that is ones that contain eggs, dairy products or nuts) – such as fruit fools, cheesecakes, egg custards or mousses and nutty biscuits – will have lower ⑤ than sugar- and carbohydrate-based ones such as wheat biscuits, chocolate cake and syrupy flapjacks. However, saturated fat should still be limited, so, if you need help to come up with some tempting puddings that still make nutritional sense, see *The Low-GL Diet Cookbook*.

PUDDINGS

GL rating	Food	Serving size in g	Looks like	GL per serving
	DAIRY PRODUCTS AND ALTERNATIVES			
1	Plain yoghurt (no sugar)	200	1 small pot	3
1	Non-fat yoghurt (plain, no sugar)	200	1 small pot	3
1	Soya yoghurt (Provamel)	200	1 large bowl	7
1	Soya milk (no sugar), in ml	250	1 glass	7
1	Custard, homemade from milk	100	1½ small cups	7
1	Low-fat yoghurt, fruit, sugar (Ski)	150	1 small pot	7.5
1	Ice cream, regular	60	2 scoops	10
	FRUIT AND FRUIT PRODUCTS			
1	Blackberries E	120	1 medium bowl	1
1	Blueberries E	120	1 medium bowl	1
1	Raspberries E	120	1 medium bowl	1
1	Strawberries, fresh, raw	120	1 medium bowl	1
1	Cherries, raw, not stoned	120	1 medium bowl	3

GL rating	Food	Serving size in g	Looks like	GL per serving
1	Grapefruit, raw	120	½ medium	3
1	Pear, raw	120	1 medium	4
1	Melon, eg cantaloupe, raw	120	½ small	4
1	Watermelon, raw	120	1 medium slice	4
1	Peaches, raw (or canned in natural juice)	120	1	5
1	Apricots, raw	120	4 apricots	5
1	Oranges, raw	120	1 large	5
1	Plums, raw	120	4	5
1	Apples, raw	120	1 small	6
1	Kiwi fruit, raw	120	1	6
1	Pineapple, raw	120	1 medium slice	7
1	Grapes, raw	120	16	8
1	Mango, raw	120	1½ slices	8
1	Apricots, dried	60	6 apricots	9
1	Fruit cocktail, canned (Delmonte)	120	small can	9
1	Pawpaw/papaya, raw	120	½ small papaya	10
1	Prunes, pitted	60	6 prunes	10

GL rating	Food	Serving size in g	Looks like	GL per serving
1	Apple, dried	60	6 rings	10
2	Banana, raw	120	1 small	12
2	Apricots, canned in light syrup	120	1 small tin	12
3	Lychees, canned in syrup and drained	120	1 small tin	16
3	Figs, dried, tenderised (Dessert Maid)	60	3	16
3	Sultanas	60	30	25
3	Raisins	60	30	28
3	Dates, dried	60	8	42
	SUGARS			
1	Xylitol	20	1 tbsp	2
1	Blue agave cactus syrup	20	1 tbsp	2
1	Fructose	20	1 tbsp	4
2	Sucrose	20	1 tbsp	14
3	Honey	20	1 tbsp	16
3	Glucose	20	1 tbsp	20
3	Maltose (malt)	20	1 tbsp	22

table continues ➤

GL rating	Food	Serving size in g	Looks like	⑤ per serving
	DESSERTS			
1	Almond custard*	–	1 serving	2
1	Tahini yoghurt*	–	1 serving	4
1	Lemon cheesecake*	–	1 slice	4
1	Blueberry/almond pancakes*	–	1 pancake	4
1	Apricot crunch*	–	1 serving	5
1	Amaretti-stuffed plums*	–	1 serving	6
1	Baked chocolate orange pots*	–	1 serving	6
1	Banana and berry frozen yoghurt*	–	1 serving	6
1	Rhubarb fool*	–	1 serving	6
1	Rice pudding*	–	1 ramekin	6
1	Pear crumble*	–	1 serving	7
1	Crème brûlée E	50	1 ramekin	10
1	Crème caramel E	50	1 ramekin	10
1	Tofu-based frozen dessert, chocolate with high fructose corn syrup (24%)	50	half an individual dessert	10
2	Chocolate hazelnut mousse*	–	1 ramekin	11
2	Chocolate mousse E	50	2 spoonfuls (small bowl)	12

GL rating	Food	Serving size in g	Looks like	GL per serving
3	Fruit crumble E	100	1 medium bowl	15
3	Fruit sorbet E	50	2 scoops	15
3	Pancake, with sugar and lemon	50	1 medium	15
3	Rice pudding	–	1 medium bowl	16
3	Cheesecake E	100	1 slice	23
3	Tiramisù E	75	1 medium bowl	25
3	Trifle E	75	1 medium bowl	25
3	Gateau E	75	1 slice	28
3	Christmas pudding E	100	1 medium bowl	30
3	Sticky toffee pudding E	100	1 medium bowl	35
3	Treacle tart E	100	1 slice	35
3	Mince pie E	100	2	50

* These items appear in *The Low-GL Diet Cookbook*
All dishes marked E have estimated GL scores

Drinks

The goal:

- have no more than 5 🔵 for drinks;

- avoid alcohol for the first two weeks when trying to lose weight in order to kick-start your weight loss;

- after the first two weeks have no more than 1 unit of alcohol per day (even if this is under 5 🔵!).

DRINKS

GL rating	Drink	Serving size in ml	Looks like	GL per serving
	DAIRY PRODUCTS AND ALTERNATIVES			
1	Milk, full-fat	250	1 glass	3
1	Milk, skim (Canada)	250	1 glass	4
1	Soya milk (no sugar)	250	1 glass	7
1	Soya milk (sweetened with apple juice concentrate)	250	1 glass	8
1	Soya milk, reduced-fat (1.5%), 120mg calcium	250	1 glass	8
1	Soya milk (sweetened with sugar)	250	1 glass	9
2	Rice milk E	250	1 glass	14
	DRINKS			
1	Lemonade*	250	1 glass	1
1	Gingerade*	250	1 glass	1
1	Strawberry smoothie*	–	1 large glass	3
1	Tomato juice, canned, no added sugar	250	½ pint	4
1	Pear and blueberry smoothie*	–	1 glass	4

table continues ➤

GL rating	Drink	Serving size in ml	Looks like	GL per serving
1	Virgin mary*	–	1 glass	4
1	Apple, lemon and ginger smoothie*	–	1 glass	5
1	Fermented milk drink with *Lactobacillus casei* (Yakult)	65	1 pot	6
1	Smoothie drink, soy, banana	250	1 individual carton	7
1	Smoothie drink, soy, chocolate, hazelnut	250	1 individual carton	8
1	Milo, dissolved in full-fat cow's milk	250	half a glass	9
1	Milo, dissolved in water	250	half a glass	9
1	Apple juice, cloudy, unsweetened	250	1 individual carton	10
1	Carrot juice, freshly made	250	1 individual carton	10
2	Grapefruit juice, unsweetened	250	1 individual carton	11
2	Apple juice, pure, unsweetened,	250	1 individual carton	12
2	Gatorade	250	half a glass	12
2	Orange juice	250	1 individual carton	13

GL rating	Drink	Serving size in ml	Looks like	GL per serving
2	Cordial, orange, reconstituted	250	1 individual carton	13
2	Smoothie, raspberry	250	1 individual carton	14
3	Pineapple juice, unsweetened	250	1 individual carton	16
3	Cranberry juice drink (Ocean Spray)	250	1 individual carton	16
3	Cola, soft drink/soda/pop	330	1 can	21
3	Orange soft drink (Fanta)	330	1 can	30
3	Lucozade, original	330	1 can	53

* These items appear in *The Low-GL Diet Cookbook*
All dishes marked E have estimated GL scores

Remember, it is not advisable to have more than 1 unit of alcohol a day, on average, or more than 5 🌀 a day if you choose to allocate all of your 5 🌀 for drinks/ desserts to an alcoholic drink. This would mean a glass of wine a day, the drier the better, or a half pint of lager every other day.

GL rating	Drink	Unit size in ml	Looks like	🌀 per serving
	ALCOHOLIC DRINKS			
1	Spirits	30	1 shot	0
1	White wine	115	1 small glass	1
1	Red wine	115	1 small glass	2
1	Spirits + orange juice	30	1 small glass	6
1	Spirits + cola	30	1 small glass	8
1	Beer/lager	300	½ pint	10

Eating Out

The goal:

- eat no more than 10 ⓖⓛ at lunch and supper to lose weight (you can also use your additional 5 ⓖⓛ for drinks or pudding here if you feel like a treat), or 15 ⓖⓛ to maintain your weight; also you can put your additional 10 ⓖⓛ towards a starter and/or pudding;

- combine protein with carbohydrate.

Although fat doesn't contain any ⓖⓛ, watch out for saturated fat in creamy sauces on curries and pasta dishes, cheese on pizzas, mayonnaise and oily salad dressings, because this is still stored as fat by the body. Better to opt for tomato-based sauces such as madras curries instead of kormas or masalas, go for extra toppings on your pizza instead of cheese and ask to dress your own salad with a little balsamic vinegar and olive oil.

Oriental food such as Thai, Vietnamese, Japanese and Korean are a good bet in terms of avoiding high-fat dairy products, and they generally use less oil for cooking and dressing food. They also tend to feature vegetables prominently, making them a very healthy choice. Don't go for the extremely high-GL white rice, sushi rice or sticky rice that accompanies most dishes, and avoid carbohydrate-heavy noodle dishes such as pad thai. You can always ask for an extra side serving of vegetables in place of the rice if you are being super-healthy, to make sure you get adequate carbohydrate, or, if you can't resist, have just a spoonful of rice or noodles.

Indian restaurants can be a dieting minefield, since, even if you avoid the creamy korma curries and the fried poppadoms, they will still cook your tomato-based curry with ghee, or clarified butter, making the saturated fat hard to avoid. Again avoid high carbohydrate naan bread and white rice.

If you think eating Italian means pizza and pasta, look at the menu more carefully next time you are out. Italian cuisine also features wonderful vegetable and meat and seafood dishes that escape being smothered in mozzarella or sprinkled with Parmesan. These make a much healthier and lower-GL choice, avoiding all that carbohydrate and saturated fat.

Lastly, just because you paid for it, or because it is put on the table, it doesn't mean you *have* to eat it. Don't accept a piece of bread before your meal arrives – or else your 7 GL carbohydrate quota is gone before you have even started! Ask for a bowl of olives instead, or, if you can't resist the smell of freshly baked bread, ask the waiter not to leave the basket on the table for you to carry on picking at, and don't have the butter.

The same goes for pudding: if you have paid for a three-course set menu but aren't particularly bothered about any of the puddings on offer, don't have one just because it is included. Think how smug you will feel tomorrow when you think that you didn't blow your GL budget. Equally, if everyone else is having a starter and you don't want to feel left out, ask for a lightly dressed mixed salad if there is nothing particularly tempting or healthy on the menu – or if you want to save your GL points for the main course or pudding.

EATING OUT

GL rating	Food	Serving size in g	Looks like	**GL** per serving
	STARTERS			
1	Beef carpaccio	30	starter portion	0
1	Moules marinières (or other sauce) E	150	starter portion	0
1	Mixed salad (dressed/ undressed)	30	starter portion	2
1	Scallops with salad E	50	starter portion	2
1	Tomato and mozzarella salad	50	starter portion	2
1	Oriental broth, such as Tom Yum soup E	–	small bowl	4
1	Sushi E	30	2 pieces fish on rice	5
1	Smoked salmon with 1 slice brown bread E	100	starter portion	10
	COMPLETE DISHES			
2	Goat's-cheese salad with 1 piece bread E	150	main-course portion	12
3	Caesar salad (with/without chicken) E	100	main-course portion	17
3	Pasta with pesto	200	large plate	18

GL rating	Food	Serving size in g	Looks like	GL per serving
3	Pizza (thin base) E	150	large slice	18
3	Pasta with cream-based sauce E	200	large plate	18
3	Lasagne E	420	large serving	20
3	Pasta with tomato-based sauce E	200	large plate	20
3	Meat with 3 large roast potatoes, carrots and gravy E	500	large plate	20
3	Risotto E	200	main-course portion	20
3	Fish/meat teriyaki/yakitori with white rice E	500	large serving	25
3	Cheeseburger E	130	medium	25
3	Hamburger E	120	medium	25
3	Fish/chicken satay (peanut sauce) with white rice E	320	medium serving	26
3	Stir-fried meat/vegetables with white rice E	350	large serving	28
3	Meat curry (cream-based sauce, such as korma, masala) with white rice E	500	large serving	28

table continues ➤

GL rating	Food	Serving size in g	Looks like	GL per serving
3	Meat curry (tomato-based sauce, such as madras, rogan josh) with white rice E	500	large serving	28
3	Meat/egg fried rice/ noodles E	350	large serving	29
3	Pizza (thick-base) E	300	large slice	36
3	Fish and chips E	550	standard takeaway portion	40
3	Garlic bread (white baguette) E	100	2 large slices	45
	PUDDINGS			
1	Custard, homemade from milk	100	1½ small cups	7
1	Ice cream, regular	60	2 scoops	10
1	Crème brûlée E	50	1 ramekin	10
1	Crème caramel E	50	1 ramekin	10
1	Chocolate mousse E	50	2 spoonfuls	10
3	Fruit crumble E	100	1 medium bowl	15
3	Fruit sorbet E	50	2 scoops	15
3	Pancake, with sugar and lemon	50	1 medium	15

GL rating	Food	Serving size in g	Looks like	Ⓖ per serving
3	Rice pudding	100	1 medium bowl	16
3	Cheesecake E	100	1 slice	23
3	Tiramisù E	75	1 medium bowl	25
3	Trifle E	75	1 medium bowl	25
3	Gateau E	75	1 slice	28
3	Christmas pudding E	100	1 medium bowl	30
3	Sticky toffee pudding E	100	1 medium bowl	35
3	Treacle tart E	100	1 slice	35
3	Mince pie E	100	2	50

All dishes marked E have estimated GL scores

Calculate Your Ⓖ Each Day

Use the chart on the next and following pages to calculate your daily GL total. Here is an example:

MEAL	TOTAL
Supper (aim = 10 Ⓖ)	
Salmon (0 Ⓖ) + rice (7 Ⓖ) + broccoli (3 Ⓖ)	10

MEAL	TOTAL
Breakfast (aim = 10 ⒼⓁ)	
Snack (aim = 5 ⒼⓁ)	
Lunch (aim = 10 ⒼⓁ)	
Snack (aim = 5 ⒼⓁ)	
Supper (aim = 10 ⒼⓁ)	
Drinks or puddings (aim = 5 ⒼⓁ)	
DAILY TOTAL	

MEAL	TOTAL
Breakfast (aim = 10 🔵)	
Snack (aim = 5 🔵)	
Lunch (aim = 10 🔵)	
Snack (aim = 5 🔵)	
Supper (aim = 10 🔵)	
Drinks or puddings (aim = 5 🔵)	
DAILY TOTAL	

MEAL	TOTAL
Breakfast (aim = 10 ⑤ⓛ)	
Snack (aim = 5 ⑤ⓛ)	
Lunch (aim = 10 ⑤ⓛ)	
Snack (aim = 5 ⑤ⓛ)	
Supper (aim = 10 ⑤ⓛ)	
Drinks or puddings (aim = 5 ⑤ⓛ)	
DAILY TOTAL	

MEAL	TOTAL
Breakfast (aim = 10 ⑥)	
Snack (aim = 5 ⑥)	
Lunch (aim = 10 ⑥)	
Snack (aim = 5 ⑥)	
Supper (aim = 10 ⑥)	
Drinks or puddings (aim = 5 ⑥)	
DAILY TOTAL	

MEAL	TOTAL
Breakfast (aim = 10 ⒢ⓛ)	
Snack (aim = 5 ⒢ⓛ)	
Lunch (aim = 10 ⒢ⓛ)	
Snack (aim = 5 ⒢ⓛ)	
Supper (aim = 10 ⒢ⓛ)	
Drinks or puddings (aim = 5 ⒢ⓛ)	
DAILY TOTAL	

MEAL	TOTAL
Breakfast (aim = 10 GL)	
Snack (aim = 5 GL)	
Lunch (aim = 10 GL)	
Snack (aim = 5 GL)	
Supper (aim = 10 GL)	
Drinks or puddings (aim = 5 GL)	
DAILY TOTAL	

MEAL	TOTAL
Breakfast (aim = 10 ⓖ)	
Snack (aim = 5 ⓖ)	
Lunch (aim = 10 ⓖ)	
Snack (aim = 5 ⓖ)	
Supper (aim = 10 ⓖ)	
Drinks or puddings (aim = 5 ⓖ)	
DAILY TOTAL	

MEAL	TOTAL
Breakfast (aim = 10 ⒼⓁ)	
Snack (aim = 5 ⒼⓁ)	
Lunch (aim = 10 ⒼⓁ)	
Snack (aim = 5 ⒼⓁ)	
Supper (aim = 10 ⒼⓁ)	
Drinks or puddings (aim = 5 ⒼⓁ)	
DAILY TOTAL	

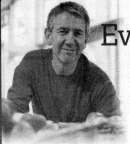

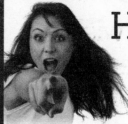

How 100% Healthy are you?

"I thought I was a healthy person. I did the online report. I feel absolutely fantastic. It's changed my life. It's amazing." Karen S

Karen before 36%

Karen after 86%

D	C	B	A
NOT GOOD	AVERAGE	REASONABLY HEALTHY	HEALTHY

YOU CAN wake up full of energy, with a clear mind and balanced mood, never gain weight and stay disease free. Having worked with over 60,000 people We know what changes are going to most rapidly transform how you feel. The **100% Health Programme** is the most comprehensive and genuinely effective way of taking a step towards 100% health.

Your **FREE Health Check** is the first step to receiving your **100% Health Programme** (£24.95), the ultimate on-line personal health profile, that shows you exactly what your perfect diet and daily supplement programme is, and which simple lifestyle changes will make the biggest difference.

You receive:

✓ A full Set of Results on your body systems and processes

✓ In-depth Report on you & your health

✓ Your Perfect Recipes and Menu Plan

✓ Your own Library of Special Reports

✓ Full Lifestyle Analysis inc:
  ▪ Exercise ▪ Stress ▪ Sleep ▪ Pollution

✓ Your Action Plan & Personal Supplement Programme;

✓ PLUS optional weekly support and guidance from Patrick;

✓ Free Reassessment to chart your progress, month by month

✓ Your questions answered by Patrick himself, plus all the benefits of membership

BEGIN YOUR **FREE** HEALTH CHECKUP NOW
Go to **www.patrickholford.com**